To use this journal simply fill in the columns:

- Time
- Type of food and how much/portion size
- Your degree of hunger from 1 -10
- Location

These details will provide insight into emotional triggers for eating habits, as well as times of day and places where healthy and unhealthy foods are most likely to be consumed.

How detailed you are is up to you. I recommend you start with just the bare basics to get in the habit and add details as you continue to log your food over the weeks. However the more thorough you are when recording what you eat (those 5 M&Ms at the office, the extra mayo on your sandwich, the sauce on your dinner) the more ways you'll eventually find to cut those extra calories. When you look back over your food diary records, look for those nibbles and bites that really do add up. Did you know that 150 extra calories in a day (that could be one beer or glass of wine or an extra splash of spread on your sandwich) could result in a 14 to 20 lb weight gain in ***one year***?

On the lined page write down anything you think is important, such as how you felt (physically and emotionally) when you finished eating, what and how much exercise you got today, any medication you have taken, and your blood sugar results, if you have diabetes.

Be aware of the common roadblocks many people face.

These are the four most common obstacles to keeping a food diary.
- Are you embarrassed or ashamed about your eating?
- Do you have a sense of hopelessness? Feeling that it won't help to fill out a food diary or that weight loss is impossible for you?
- Does it seem too inconvenient to write down what you eat/drink?
- Do you feel bad when you "slip up"?

What's the cure?

- All of these roadblocks can be overcome by remembering the usefulness of the journals
- Not trying to be perfect
- Knowing that slips will happen
- And staying motivated to use tools that promote health and well-being

Date:

Time	Food & Portion Size	Hunger	Location

Water ☐ ☐ ☐ ☐ ☐ ☐ ☐ ☐ ☐ ☐ ☐

Date:

Time	Food & Portion Size	Hunger	Location
Water	☐ ☐ ☐ ☐ ☐ ☐ ☐ ☐ ☐ ☐ ☐		

Date:

Time	Food & Portion Size	Hunger	Location

Water ☐ ☐ ☐ ☐ ☐ ☐ ☐ ☐ ☐ ☐ ☐

Date:

Time	Food & Portion Size	Hunger	Location

Water ☐ ☐ ☐ ☐ ☐ ☐ ☐ ☐ ☐ ☐ ☐

Date:

Time	Food & Portion Size	Hunger	Location
Water	☐ ☐ ☐ ☐ ☐ ☐ ☐ ☐ ☐ ☐ ☐		

Date:

Time	Food & Portion Size	Hunger	Location

Water	☐ ☐ ☐ ☐ ☐ ☐ ☐ ☐ ☐ ☐ ☐

Date:

Time	Food & Portion Size	Hunger	Location

Water	☐ ☐ ☐ ☐ ☐ ☐ ☐ ☐ ☐ ☐

Date:

Time	Food & Portion Size	Hunger	Location

Water ☐ ☐ ☐ ☐ ☐ ☐ ☐ ☐ ☐ ☐ ☐

Date:

Time	Food & Portion Size	Hunger	Location

Water ☐ ☐ ☐ ☐ ☐ ☐ ☐ ☐ ☐ ☐ ☐

Date:

Time	Food & Portion Size	Hunger	Location

Water   ☐ ☐ ☐ ☐ ☐ ☐ ☐ ☐ ☐ ☐ ☐

Date:

Time	Food & Portion Size	Hunger	Location

Water ☐ ☐ ☐ ☐ ☐ ☐ ☐ ☐ ☐ ☐ ☐

Date:

Time	Food & Portion Size	Hunger	Location

Water ☐ ☐ ☐ ☐ ☐ ☐ ☐ ☐ ☐ ☐ ☐

Date:

Time	Food & Portion Size	Hunger	Location

Water ☐ ☐ ☐ ☐ ☐ ☐ ☐ ☐ ☐ ☐ ☐

Date:

Time	Food & Portion Size	Hunger	Location

Water	☐ ☐ ☐ ☐ ☐ ☐ ☐ ☐ ☐ ☐ ☐

Date:

Time	Food & Portion Size	Hunger	Location

Water ☐ ☐ ☐ ☐ ☐ ☐ ☐ ☐ ☐ ☐ ☐

Date:

Time	Food & Portion Size	Hunger	Location
Water	☐ ☐ ☐ ☐ ☐ ☐ ☐ ☐ ☐ ☐ ☐		

Date:

Time	Food & Portion Size	Hunger	Location

Water ☐ ☐ ☐ ☐ ☐ ☐ ☐ ☐ ☐ ☐ ☐

Date:

Time	Food & Portion Size	Hunger	Location

Water ☐ ☐ ☐ ☐ ☐ ☐ ☐ ☐ ☐ ☐ ☐

Date:

Time	Food & Portion Size	Hunger	Location
Water	☐ ☐ ☐ ☐ ☐ ☐ ☐ ☐ ☐ ☐ ☐		

Date:

Time	Food & Portion Size	Hunger	Location

Water ☐ ☐ ☐ ☐ ☐ ☐ ☐ ☐ ☐ ☐ ☐

Date:

Time	Food & Portion Size	Hunger	Location

Water ☐ ☐ ☐ ☐ ☐ ☐ ☐ ☐ ☐ ☐ ☐

Date:

Time	Food & Portion Size	Hunger	Location
Water	☐ ☐ ☐ ☐ ☐ ☐ ☐ ☐ ☐ ☐ ☐		

Date:

Time	Food & Portion Size	Hunger	Location

Water ☐ ☐ ☐ ☐ ☐ ☐ ☐ ☐ ☐ ☐ ☐

Date:

Time	Food & Portion Size	Hunger	Location

Water	☐ ☐ ☐ ☐ ☐ ☐ ☐ ☐ ☐ ☐ ☐

Date:

Time	Food & Portion Size	Hunger	Location
Water	☐ ☐ ☐ ☐ ☐ ☐ ☐ ☐ ☐ ☐ ☐		

Date:

Time	Food & Portion Size	Hunger	Location

Water ☐ ☐ ☐ ☐ ☐ ☐ ☐ ☐ ☐ ☐ ☐

Date:

Time	Food & Portion Size	Hunger	Location

Water ☐ ☐ ☐ ☐ ☐ ☐ ☐ ☐ ☐ ☐ ☐

Date:

Time	Food & Portion Size	Hunger	Location

Water ☐ ☐ ☐ ☐ ☐ ☐ ☐ ☐ ☐ ☐ ☐

Date:

Time	Food & Portion Size	Hunger	Location

Water ☐ ☐ ☐ ☐ ☐ ☐ ☐ ☐ ☐ ☐ ☐

Date:

Time	Food & Portion Size	Hunger	Location

Water ☐ ☐ ☐ ☐ ☐ ☐ ☐ ☐ ☐ ☐ ☐

Date:

Time	Food & Portion Size	Hunger	Location

Water ☐ ☐ ☐ ☐ ☐ ☐ ☐ ☐ ☐ ☐ ☐

Date:

Time	Food & Portion Size	Hunger	Location
Water	☐ ☐ ☐ ☐ ☐ ☐ ☐ ☐ ☐ ☐ ☐		

Date:

Time	Food & Portion Size	Hunger	Location

Water ☐ ☐ ☐ ☐ ☐ ☐ ☐ ☐ ☐ ☐ ☐

Date:

Time	Food & Portion Size	Hunger	Location
Water	☐ ☐ ☐ ☐ ☐ ☐ ☐ ☐ ☐ ☐ ☐		

Date:

Time	Food & Portion Size	Hunger	Location

Water ☐ ☐ ☐ ☐ ☐ ☐ ☐ ☐ ☐ ☐ ☐

Date:

Time	Food & Portion Size	Hunger	Location

Water ☐ ☐ ☐ ☐ ☐ ☐ ☐ ☐ ☐ ☐ ☐

Date:

Time	Food & Portion Size	Hunger	Location

Water ☐ ☐ ☐ ☐ ☐ ☐ ☐ ☐ ☐ ☐ ☐

Date:

Time	Food & Portion Size	Hunger	Location

Water ☐ ☐ ☐ ☐ ☐ ☐ ☐ ☐ ☐ ☐ ☐

Date:

Time	Food & Portion Size	Hunger	Location

Water	☐ ☐ ☐ ☐ ☐ ☐ ☐ ☐ ☐ ☐ ☐

Date:

Time	Food & Portion Size	Hunger	Location

Water   ☐ ☐ ☐ ☐ ☐ ☐ ☐ ☐ ☐ ☐ ☐

Date:

Time	Food & Portion Size	Hunger	Location

Water ☐ ☐ ☐ ☐ ☐ ☐ ☐ ☐ ☐ ☐ ☐

Date:

Time	Food & Portion Size	Hunger	Location

Water ☐ ☐ ☐ ☐ ☐ ☐ ☐ ☐ ☐ ☐ ☐

Date:

Time	Food & Portion Size	Hunger	Location

Water	☐ ☐ ☐ ☐ ☐ ☐ ☐ ☐ ☐ ☐ ☐

Date:

Time	Food & Portion Size	Hunger	Location
Water	☐ ☐ ☐ ☐ ☐ ☐ ☐ ☐ ☐ ☐		

Date:

Time	Food & Portion Size	Hunger	Location
Water	☐ ☐ ☐ ☐ ☐ ☐ ☐ ☐ ☐ ☐ ☐		

Date:

Time	Food & Portion Size	Hunger	Location

Water ☐ ☐ ☐ ☐ ☐ ☐ ☐ ☐ ☐ ☐ ☐

Date:

Time	Food & Portion Size	Hunger	Location

Water	☐ ☐ ☐ ☐ ☐ ☐ ☐ ☐ ☐ ☐

Date:

Time	Food & Portion Size	Hunger	Location
Water	☐ ☐ ☐ ☐ ☐ ☐ ☐ ☐ ☐ ☐ ☐		

Date:

Time	Food & Portion Size	Hunger	Location

Water ☐ ☐ ☐ ☐ ☐ ☐ ☐ ☐ ☐ ☐ ☐

Date:

Time	Food & Portion Size	Hunger	Location
Water	☐ ☐ ☐ ☐ ☐ ☐ ☐ ☐ ☐ ☐ ☐		

Date:

Time	Food & Portion Size	Hunger	Location

Water ☐ ☐ ☐ ☐ ☐ ☐ ☐ ☐ ☐ ☐ ☐

Date:

Time	Food & Portion Size	Hunger	Location

Water ☐ ☐ ☐ ☐ ☐ ☐ ☐ ☐ ☐ ☐ ☐

Date:

Time	Food & Portion Size	Hunger	Location

Water ☐ ☐ ☐ ☐ ☐ ☐ ☐ ☐ ☐ ☐ ☐

Date:

Time	Food & Portion Size	Hunger	Location

Water ☐ ☐ ☐ ☐ ☐ ☐ ☐ ☐ ☐ ☐ ☐

Date:

Time	Food & Portion Size	Hunger	Location
Water	☐ ☐ ☐ ☐ ☐ ☐ ☐ ☐ ☐ ☐ ☐		

Date:

Time	Food & Portion Size	Hunger	Location

Water ☐ ☐ ☐ ☐ ☐ ☐ ☐ ☐ ☐ ☐ ☐

Date:

Time	Food & Portion Size	Hunger	Location
Water	☐ ☐ ☐ ☐ ☐ ☐ ☐ ☐ ☐ ☐ ☐		

Date:

Time	Food & Portion Size	Hunger	Location

Water ☐ ☐ ☐ ☐ ☐ ☐ ☐ ☐ ☐ ☐ ☐

Date:

Time	Food & Portion Size	Hunger	Location

Water ☐ ☐ ☐ ☐ ☐ ☐ ☐ ☐ ☐ ☐

Date:

Time	Food & Portion Size	Hunger	Location
Water	☐ ☐ ☐ ☐ ☐ ☐ ☐ ☐ ☐ ☐		

Date:

Time	Food & Portion Size	Hunger	Location

Water ☐ ☐ ☐ ☐ ☐ ☐ ☐ ☐ ☐ ☐ ☐

Date:

Time	Food & Portion Size	Hunger	Location

Water ☐ ☐ ☐ ☐ ☐ ☐ ☐ ☐ ☐ ☐ ☐

Date:

Time	Food & Portion Size	Hunger	Location
Water	☐ ☐ ☐ ☐ ☐ ☐ ☐ ☐ ☐ ☐ ☐		

Date:

Time	Food & Portion Size	Hunger	Location
Water	☐ ☐ ☐ ☐ ☐ ☐ ☐ ☐ ☐ ☐ ☐		

Date:

Time	Food & Portion Size	Hunger	Location

Water ☐ ☐ ☐ ☐ ☐ ☐ ☐ ☐ ☐ ☐

Date:

Time	Food & Portion Size	Hunger	Location

Water ☐ ☐ ☐ ☐ ☐ ☐ ☐ ☐ ☐ ☐ ☐

Date:

Time	Food & Portion Size	Hunger	Location

Water ☐ ☐ ☐ ☐ ☐ ☐ ☐ ☐ ☐ ☐ ☐

Date:

Time	Food & Portion Size	Hunger	Location

Water ☐ ☐ ☐ ☐ ☐ ☐ ☐ ☐ ☐ ☐

Date:

Time	Food & Portion Size	Hunger	Location

Water ☐ ☐ ☐ ☐ ☐ ☐ ☐ ☐ ☐ ☐ ☐

Date:

Time	Food & Portion Size	Hunger	Location
Water	☐ ☐ ☐ ☐ ☐ ☐ ☐ ☐ ☐ ☐ ☐		

Date:

Time	Food & Portion Size	Hunger	Location

Water ☐ ☐ ☐ ☐ ☐ ☐ ☐ ☐ ☐ ☐ ☐

Date:

Time	Food & Portion Size	Hunger	Location

Water ☐ ☐ ☐ ☐ ☐ ☐ ☐ ☐ ☐ ☐ ☐

Date:

Time	Food & Portion Size	Hunger	Location

Water ☐ ☐ ☐ ☐ ☐ ☐ ☐ ☐ ☐ ☐ ☐

Date:

Time	Food & Portion Size	Hunger	Location

Water	☐ ☐ ☐ ☐ ☐ ☐ ☐ ☐ ☐ ☐

Date:

Time	Food & Portion Size	Hunger	Location
Water	☐ ☐ ☐ ☐ ☐ ☐ ☐ ☐ ☐ ☐ ☐		

Date:

Time	Food & Portion Size	Hunger	Location
Water	☐ ☐ ☐ ☐ ☐ ☐ ☐ ☐ ☐ ☐		

Date:

Time	Food & Portion Size	Hunger	Location

Water ☐ ☐ ☐ ☐ ☐ ☐ ☐ ☐ ☐ ☐ ☐

Date:

Time	Food & Portion Size	Hunger	Location

Water	☐ ☐ ☐ ☐ ☐ ☐ ☐ ☐ ☐ ☐ ☐

Date:

Time	Food & Portion Size	Hunger	Location

Water ☐ ☐ ☐ ☐ ☐ ☐ ☐ ☐ ☐ ☐ ☐

Date:

Time	Food & Portion Size	Hunger	Location

Water	☐ ☐ ☐ ☐ ☐ ☐ ☐ ☐ ☐ ☐ ☐

Date:

Time	Food & Portion Size	Hunger	Location

Water ☐ ☐ ☐ ☐ ☐ ☐ ☐ ☐ ☐ ☐ ☐

Date:

Time	Food & Portion Size	Hunger	Location

Water ☐ ☐ ☐ ☐ ☐ ☐ ☐ ☐ ☐ ☐ ☐

Date:

Time	Food & Portion Size	Hunger	Location

Water ☐ ☐ ☐ ☐ ☐ ☐ ☐ ☐ ☐ ☐ ☐

Date:

Time	Food & Portion Size	Hunger	Location
Water	☐ ☐ ☐ ☐ ☐ ☐ ☐ ☐ ☐ ☐ ☐		

Date:

Time	Food & Portion Size	Hunger	Location
Water	☐ ☐ ☐ ☐ ☐ ☐ ☐ ☐ ☐ ☐ ☐		

Date:

Time	Food & Portion Size	Hunger	Location

Water ☐ ☐ ☐ ☐ ☐ ☐ ☐ ☐ ☐ ☐ ☐

Date:

Time	Food & Portion Size	Hunger	Location

Water ☐ ☐ ☐ ☐ ☐ ☐ ☐ ☐ ☐ ☐ ☐

Date:

Time	Food & Portion Size	Hunger	Location
Water	☐ ☐ ☐ ☐ ☐ ☐ ☐ ☐ ☐ ☐ ☐		

Date:

Time	Food & Portion Size	Hunger	Location
Water	☐ ☐ ☐ ☐ ☐ ☐ ☐ ☐ ☐ ☐ ☐		

Date:

Time	Food & Portion Size	Hunger	Location

Water	☐ ☐ ☐ ☐ ☐ ☐ ☐ ☐ ☐ ☐ ☐

Date:

Time	Food & Portion Size	Hunger	Location

Water ☐ ☐ ☐ ☐ ☐ ☐ ☐ ☐ ☐ ☐ ☐

Date:

Time	Food & Portion Size	Hunger	Location
Water	☐ ☐ ☐ ☐ ☐ ☐ ☐ ☐ ☐ ☐ ☐		

Date:

Time	Food & Portion Size	Hunger	Location
Water	☐ ☐ ☐ ☐ ☐ ☐ ☐ ☐ ☐ ☐ ☐		

Date:

Time	Food & Portion Size	Hunger	Location
Water	☐ ☐ ☐ ☐ ☐ ☐ ☐ ☐ ☐ ☐ ☐		

Date:

Time	Food & Portion Size	Hunger	Location

Water ☐ ☐ ☐ ☐ ☐ ☐ ☐ ☐ ☐ ☐ ☐

Date:

Time	Food & Portion Size	Hunger	Location

Water ☐ ☐ ☐ ☐ ☐ ☐ ☐ ☐ ☐ ☐ ☐

Date:

Time	Food & Portion Size	Hunger	Location

Water	□ □ □ □ □ □ □ □ □ □ □

Date:

Time	Food & Portion Size	Hunger	Location

Water ☐ ☐ ☐ ☐ ☐ ☐ ☐ ☐ ☐ ☐ ☐

Date:

Time	Food & Portion Size	Hunger	Location
Water	☐ ☐ ☐ ☐ ☐ ☐ ☐ ☐ ☐ ☐ ☐		

AMAZING!

You made it to the end of this journal!

Now take a few minutes to look back and see how far you have come and celebrate that **_you did it!_**

Congratulations on all your success and sticking with it but this isn't the end of the journey. Keep logging your food every day to ensure you keep those pounds from creeping back!

-- Trish Vroom

www.ingramcontent.com/pod-product-compliance
Lightning Source LLC
Chambersburg PA
CBHW051257250726
48656CB00004B/1331